Vegetarian Recipes for Beginners

A comprehensive cookbook on the plant-based diet. Discover how to quickly and easily prepare delicious dishes, while eating healthy and without sacrificing taste!

Tasty Veggie

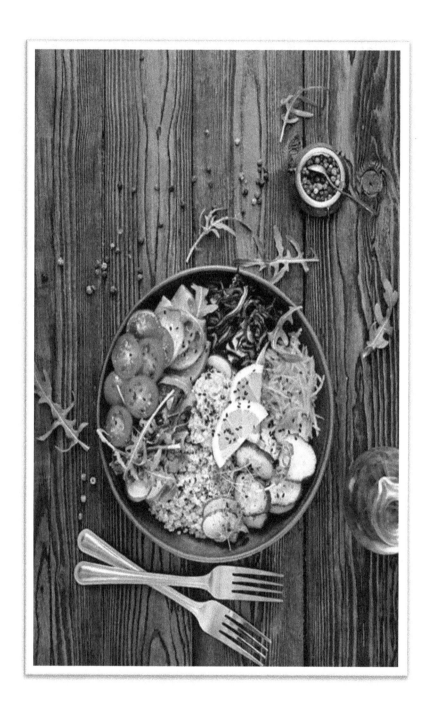

Furthermore, the transmission, duplication, or reproduction of any of the following work including specific information will be considered an illegal act irrespective of if it is done electronically or in print. This extends to creating a secondary or tertiary copy of the work or a recorded copy and is only allowed with the express written consent from the Publisher.

All additional right reserved.

The information in the following pages is broadly considered a truthful and accurate account of facts and as such, any inattention, use, or misuse of the information in question by the reader will render any resulting actions solely under their purview. There are no scenarios in which the publisher or the original author of this work can be in any fashion.

Table of Contents

INTRODUCTION

Vegetarians also need to eat a balanced and healthy diet to provide themselves with essential nutrients. A vegetarian food pyramid gives a detailed overview of all the necessary food groups. Vegetarians should include the following foods in their diet in a varied way.

WATER

At the very bottom, and thus the basis of the vegetarian food pyramid, are water and unsweetened drinks (e.g., tea). Everyone should drink 1–2 liters of water a day.

FRUIT AND VEGETABLES

In second place are fruits and vegetables. Everyone - whether vegetarian or not - should eat around 5 servings a day. In the best case, 3 servings of vegetables and 2 servings of fruit. One serving corresponds to a handful.

CEREALS AND POTATOES

The third level of the vegetarian food pyramid is cereals and potatoes. They provide us with a lot of energy and essential nutrients through carbohydrates, protein, vitamins, and fiber. In the best-case scenario, use whole grain products instead of wheat products. We recommend a total of 2–3 servings of cereals and potatoes a day.

LEGUMES AND PROTEIN PRODUCTS

The next level is of particular importance for vegetarians because legumes, soy products & Co. are essential sources of protein instead of meat and fish. Peas, lentils, beans, tofu, tempeh, and soy milk can be integrated into the menu in many ways, preferably 1–2 servings a week.

NUTS AND SEEDS

Seeds and nuts are also rich in protein and healthy fats. Almonds, walnuts, sesame, or flax seeds are suitable for snacking or refining salads and soups. 30 to 60 g a day is ideal.

FATS & OILS

Omega-3 fats such as flax, walnut, or hemp oil are particularly healthy. However, these should never be heated above 42 ° C. It is safer for frying z: B. coconut oil or sunflower oil. In general, you should consume around 2–4 tablespoons a day.

DAIRY PRODUCTS

Vegetarians who do not do without milk and dairy products - except ovo vegetarians (see above) - are allowed to eat cheese, yogurt, and quark. We recommend up to 250 ml milk or up to 50 g cheese per day.

EGGS

Everyone should eat 2 eggs a week. The so-called lacto-vegetarians (see above) are excluded because they do without eggs and products made from eggs.

SNACKS, ALCOHOL & SWEETS

Wine, chips, gummy bears & Co. form the top of the vegetarian food pyramid and should only be consumed in moderation.

VEGETARIAN BREAKFAST RECIPES

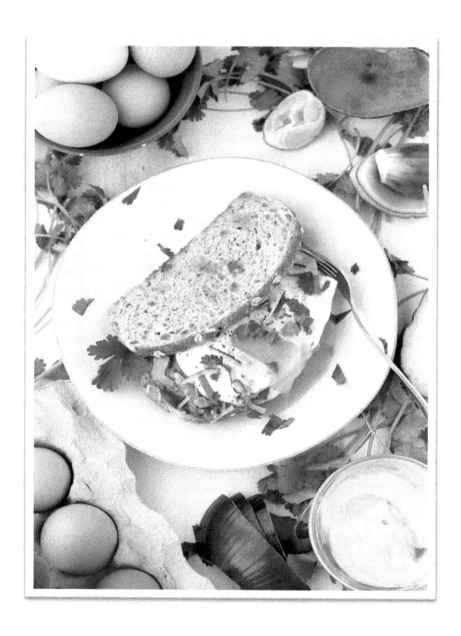

BARLEY PORRIDGE

Servings:4

INGREDIENTS

- ✓ 1 Cup barley
- ✓ 2 Schb Ginger
- ✓ 2 Pc Cardamom pods
- ✓ 1 Prize Salt
- ✓ 250 g Seasonal berries
- ✓ 1 Tbsp Sunflower seeds
- ✓ 1 Tbsp Cocoa powder
- ✓ 4 Bl Mint
- ✓ 1 Cup water

PREPARATION

1. Put one cup of barley in a saucepan with 10 cups of water.
2. Add the ginger and cardamom pods, bring to the boil, put the lid on, and cook the saucepan on a low flame for about 2 hours.
3. Put the barley porridge in a bowl and mix with the sunflower seeds, cocoa powder, and salt pinch. Fold fresh berries into the pulp and sprinkle with fresh mint.

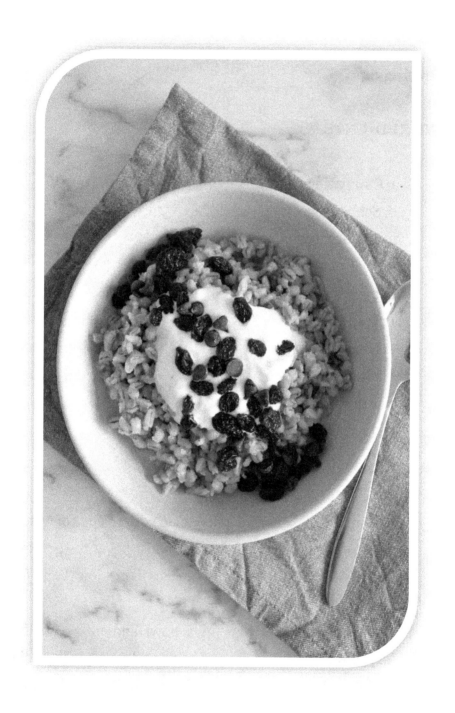

FRIED EGGS WITH CHEESE

Servings:2

INGREDIENTS

- ✓ 2 Pc Eggs
- ✓ 2 Tl Olive oil
- ✓ 2 Schb cheese
- ✓ 1 Prize Oregano
- ✓ 1 Prize Pepper
- ✓ 1 Prize Salt

PREPARATION

1. Whip the eggs in a cup, cut the cheese into strips, heat the olive oil in a pan, and add the eggs to the pan.
2. Spread the cheese on the egg whites and cover and fry until the cheese has melted and the yolk is a bit thick.
3. Slide the fried eggs onto a plate and serve sprinkled with oregano.

RADISH SPREAD

Servings:4

INGREDIENTS

- ✓ 1 Federation radish
- ✓ 1 Tbsp Sour cream
- ✓ 250 g Potting
- ✓ 1 Prize Pepper
- ✓ 1 Prize Salt

PREPARATION

1. Finely grate the radishes, squeeze out the water by hand, and place in a bowl.
2. Season to taste with curd, cream, salt, and pepper.

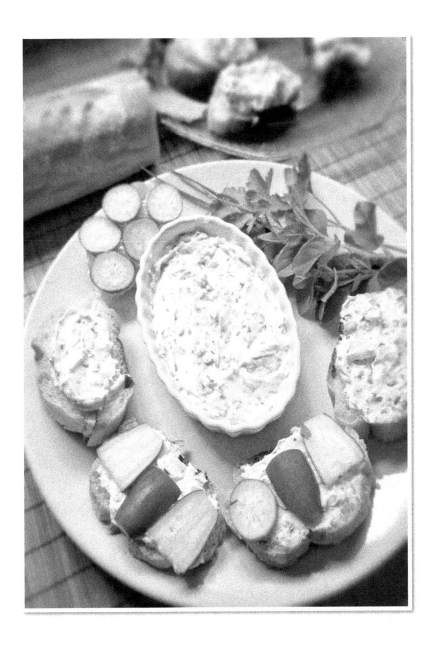

PUMPKIN SEED BREAD

Servings:1

INGREDIENTS

- ✓ 400 g Wheat flour (type 550)
- ✓ 120 g Pumpkin seeds
- ✓ 350 ml Water
- ✓ 20 g Germ
- ✓ 4 Tl Sesame
- ✓ 4 Tbsp Pumpkin seed oil
- ✓ 1 Tl Coriander
- ✓ 1 Prize Salt
- ✓ 100 g Rye flour (type 1150)

PREPARATION

1. Roast the pumpkin seeds dry, and chill. Warm water to 25 ° C. Mix in the yeast, flour, spices, and sesame seeds.
2. Add the pumpkin seeds and pumpkin seed oil to the mixture, mix well and knead.
3. Let the dough rise 2-3 times for 40 minutes each time, shape into a roll, and let it rise in the loaf pan for another 30 minutes.

4. Bake at 220 ° C top and bottom heat (preheated) for about 30 minutes, and after switching off, leave in the oven for about 10 minutes.

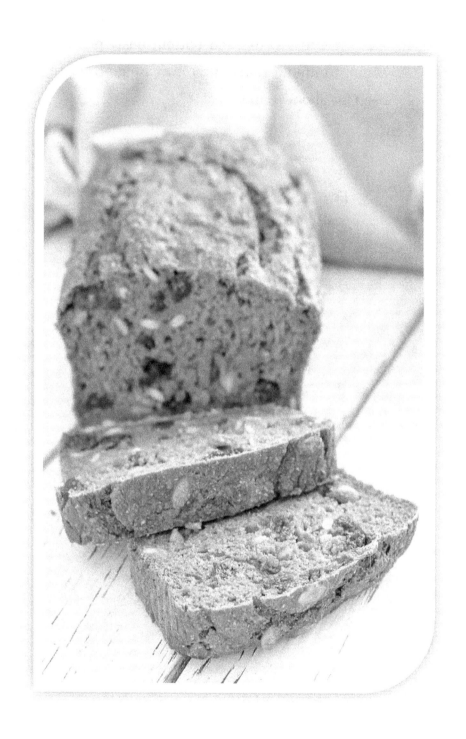

VEGETARIAN EGG SPREAD

Servings:10

INGREDIENTS

- ✓ 4 Pc Eggs
- ✓ 50 g Butter
- ✓ 1 Tbsp Mayonnaise
- ✓ 7 Pc Pickles
- ✓ 2 Pc Garlic cloves
- ✓ 2 Pc Onions
- ✓ 1 Prize Salt
- ✓ 1 Prize Pepper
- ✓ 1 Tl Mustard

PREPARATION

1. First, the hard-boiled eggs, onions and pickles, and garlic are cut into small pieces and mixed.
2. Now you just have to mix the butter with the mayonnaise and the mustard and add it to the eggs. In the end, everything is stirred vigorously until everything is well distributed and seasoned with salt and pepper and best served with fresh bread.

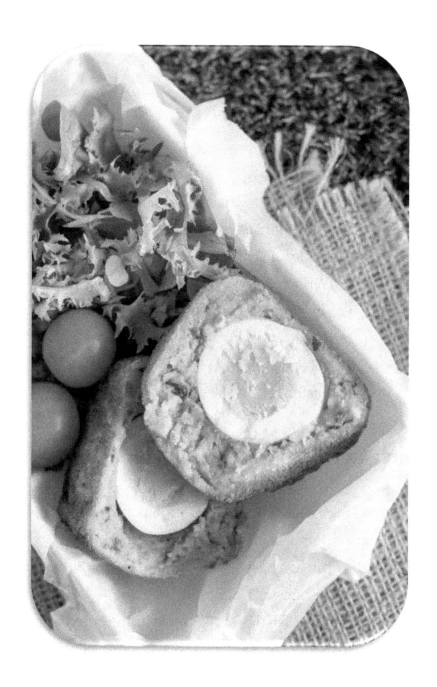

KERNEL OIL SPREAD

Servings:20

INGREDIENTS

- ✓ 1 Cups Creme fraiche Cheese
- ✓ 1 Cups Gervais
- ✓ 5 Tbsp Pumpkin seed oil
- ✓ 1 Prize Salt
- ✓ 1 Prize Pepper
- ✓ 2 Pc Garlic cloves, pressed
- ✓ 100 g Pumpkin seeds
- ✓ 1 Pc Egg

PREPARATION

1. Mix the ingredients creme fraiche, gervais, pumpkin seed oil, salt, pepper, pressed garlic, pumpkin seeds, and whisked egg together.

WHEAT GERM MUESLI

Servings:2

INGREDIENTS

- ✓ 2 Cups Organic buttermilk
- ✓ 2 Tbsp Linseed
- ✓ 2 Tbsp Lactose
- ✓ 2 Tbsp Whole sea buckthorn fruit
- ✓ 2 Tbsp Wheat germ

PREPARATION

1. Mix organic yogurt with whole sea buckthorn fruit, add lactose, and flaxseed. Sprinkle with wheat germ and serve.

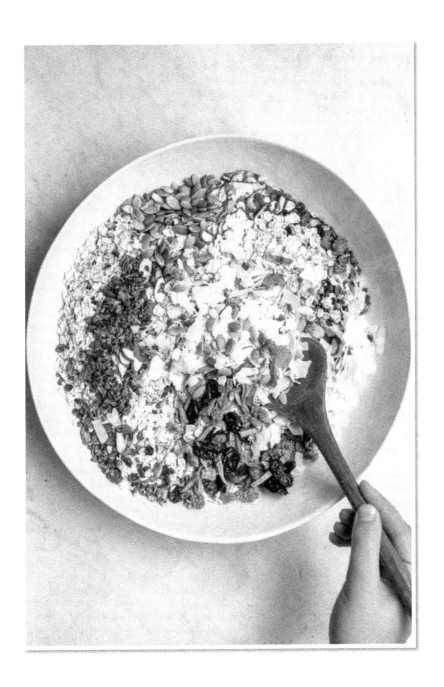

APPLE JAM

Servings:1

INGREDIENTS

- ✓ 1 Pc Lemon
- ✓ 0.5 Fl Gelling agent
- ✓ 1 kg Tart apples
- ✓ 1 kg Sugar
- ✓ 0.5 l Water

PREPARATION

1. Rub the lemon peel and squeeze the lemon.
2. Peel and core the apples, cut into small cubes, and drizzle with a bit of lemon juice.
3. Bring about 1/2 liter of water with lemon juice, zest, and sugar to the boil, add the apple pieces, stir in the gelling agent and bring to the boil until it is bubbly. Pour hot into jars and close.

VEGETARIAN LUNCH RECIPES

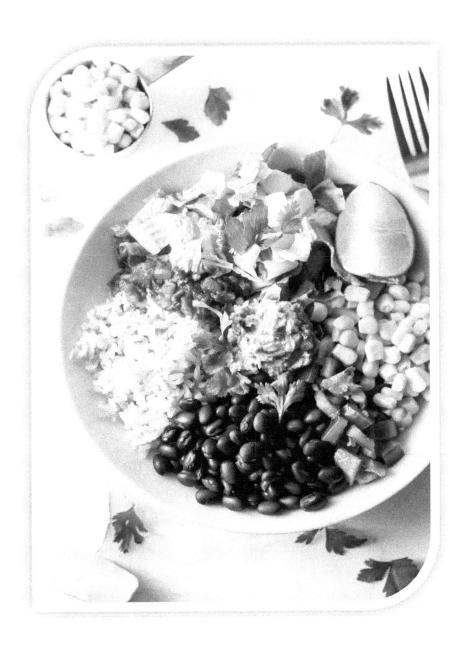

RAFFAELLO

Servings:20

INGREDIENTS

- ✓ 110 g Icing sugar
- ✓ 2 Pk vanilla sugar
- ✓ 100 g Butter
- ✓ 330 g White chocolate (finely grated)
- ✓ 1 Shot Rum
- ✓ 5 Tbsp Orange juice
- ✓ 150 g Desiccated coconut
- ✓ 5 Tbsp Desiccated coconut for rolling

PREPARATION

1. For the homemade Raffaello balls, whip the butter with the icing sugar and vanilla sugar in a bowl until frothy.
2. Now add a dash of rum (you can leave it out), white chocolate, orange juice, and coconut flakes, and knead the mixture well.
3. This is used to form small, bite-sized balls - if you want, you can also add a small piece of nut or a peeled almond to the ball.

4. Just roll in coconut flakes, and the homemade Raffaello balls are ready.

WOK VEGETABLES

Servings:4

INGREDIENTS

- ✓ 200 g Green beans
- ✓ 1 Prize Pepper
- ✓ 2 Pc Onion
- ✓ 10 Pc Broccoli
- ✓ 1 Pc Chilli Pepper
- ✓ 1 Tbsp Toasted sesame seeds
- ✓ 1 Tl Dark sauce thickener
- ✓ 3 Tbsp Hoisin or soy sauce
- ✓ 200 ml Vegetable broth
- ✓ 3 Tbsp Sesame oil
- ✓ 200 g Red pepper
- ✓ 1 Prize Salt

PREPARATION

1. Clean the beans and cook in salted water for 5 minutes, drain and drain. Halve the onion and cut it into half rings. Core and finely chop the chili pepper. Clean the

pepper and cut it into strips. Wash the broccoli and add to the wok as well.

2. Heat the sesame oil in a wok or a non-stick pan, add the vegetables and chili and fry for 3 minutes. Deglaze with vegetable stock and cook for 3-4 minutes over medium heat. Season with salt, pepper, and hoisin sauce (or soy sauce). Stir in the sauce thickener, bring to the boil. Sprinkle with toasted sesame seeds

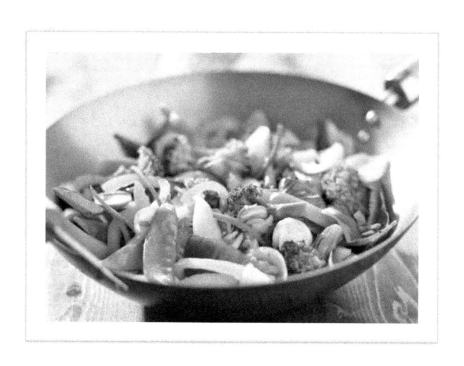

CLASSIC COCKTAIL SAUCE

Servings:4

INGREDIENTS

- ✓ 1 Shot Brandy (or cognac)
- ✓ 2 Tbsp Ketchup
- ✓ 1 Tbsp Mayonnaise (easy)
- ✓ 2 Tbsp Whipped cream
- ✓ 1 Prize Salt
- ✓ 1 Msp Pepper White
- ✓ 0.5 Cups Yogurt
- ✓ 1 Prize Chilli powder
- ✓ 1 Prize Sugar

PREPARATION

1. For this quick cocktail sauce, mix the yogurt with tomato ketchup, mayonnaise, cream, and a dash of brandy in a bowl.
2. Season the sauce with salt, pepper, sugar, and chili powder as desired.

ZUCCHINI PATTIES

Servings:4

INGREDIENTS

- ✓ 4 Pc Zucchini
- ✓ 4 Pc Potatoes
- ✓ 2 Pc Onions
- ✓ 1 Prize Salt
- ✓ 4 Tbsp Oil
- ✓ 1 Pc Egg
- ✓ 3 Tbsp Flour, for turning
- ✓ 50 g Flour, for the mass
- ✓ 3 Tbsp Basil, chopped

PREPARATION

1. Peel the zucchini and potatoes, grate with a grater and squeeze the whole thing well.
2. Now finely chop the onions and stir into the potato-zucchini mixture.
3. Season with salt, pepper, and any herbs (e.g., dill, garlic, basil) and stir well.

4. Finally, stir in the egg and flour, leave it to stand for about 15 minutes and then form patties out of them - turn them in flour.

5. Heat the oil in a pan and fry the raw zucchini patties on both sides for about 3-5 minutes.

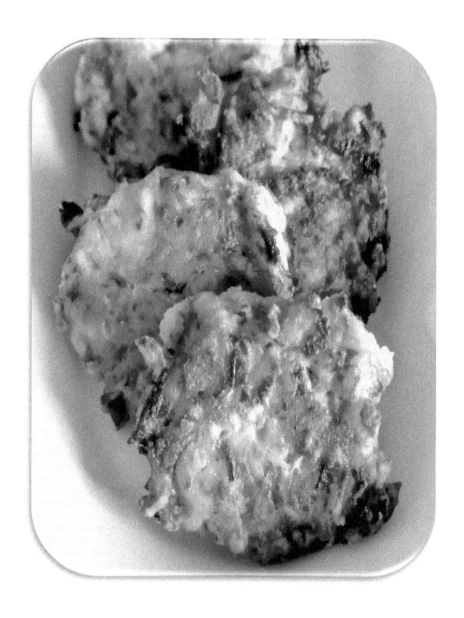

POT DUMPLINGS WITH BREADCRUMBS

Servings:4

INGREDIENTS

- ✓ 1 Cups Curd cheese (fine, 250 g)
- ✓ 1 Pc Eggs
- ✓ 1 Prize Salt
- ✓ 3 Tbsp Flour
- ✓ 3 Tbsp Semolina
- ✓ 3 Tbsp Butter
- ✓ 3 Tbsp Crumbs
- ✓ 1 Tbsp Sugar

PREPARATION

1. For the pot dumplings with crumbs, first work the curd, egg, flour, semolina, and salt into a smooth dough, then leave to rest for 10 minutes.
2. In the meantime, bring a saucepan of salted water to the boil and use two spoons to form dumplings from the dough. Let the dumplings simmer in boiling water for about 15 minutes.

3. In the meantime, melt the butter in a pan, add the crumbs and sugar, and toast. Lift the dumplings out of the water with the slotted spoon and roll them in the butter crumbs.

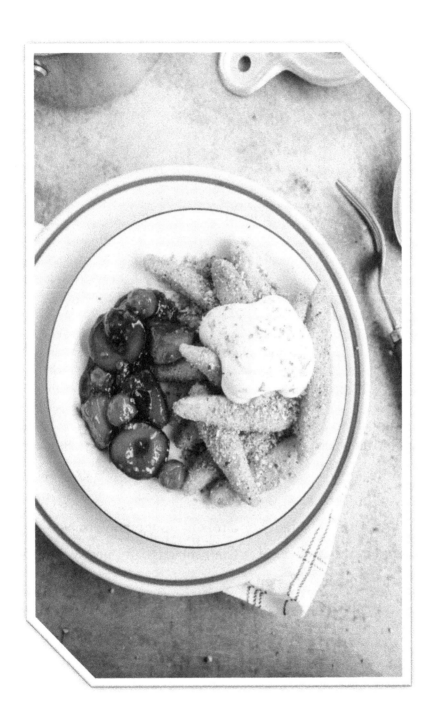

SPAETZLE BASE DOUGH

Servings:4

INGREDIENTS

- ✓ 3 Pc Eggs
- ✓ 1 Prize Salt for the saltwater
- ✓ 130 ml water
- ✓ 300 g Wheat flour
- ✓ 1 Tbsp Butter
- ✓ 1 Tl Salt

PREPARATION

1. Put the wheat flour in a bowl. Make a well in the middle of the wheat flour with a spoon and add the eggs, water 130 ml, and salt.

2. Either use your hand or a mixer/dough hook to beat the dough until it separates from the edge of the bowl and a thick dough is formed.

3. Cover the dough in the bowl with a kitchen towel and let it rest in a warm place for about 30-45 minutes.

4. Then bring a (large) pot of salted water to the boil and slowly slide the spaetzle into the boiling water with the help of a spaetzle slicer or a spaetzle sieve.

5. Cook the spaetzle until they come up and float on the surface. It is best to remove the spaetzle with a slotted spoon.

6. Now you can briefly toast the finished spaetzle in a pan with hot butter and serve immediately.

CARROT SALAD

Servings:4

INGREDIENTS

- ✓ 400 g Carrots
- ✓ 1 TL honey
- ✓ 0.5 Pc Lemon, juice

For the Vinaigrette
- 1 Shot Oil
- 100 ml water
- 0.5 Tl Salt
- 1 Shot Vinegar (light of your choice)

PREPARATION

1. For the carrot salad, brush and wash the carrots, grate them finely, season with honey and lemon juice.
2. Only the oil on top and the vinaigrette. The vinaigrette is made from water, salt, and vinegar.
3. Let stand for at least 30 minutes.

SPINACH LASAGNE WITH BECHAMEL SAUCE

Servings:4

INGREDIENTS

- ✓ 2 Pc Onion
- ✓ 4 Pc Garlic cloves
- ✓ 600 g Spinach - TK
- ✓ 1 Msp Nutmeg
- ✓ 250 g Feta
- ✓ 120 g Cheese (grated)
- ✓ 16 Pc Lasagna sheets
- ✓ 1 Tbsp Oil for the mold
- ✓ 2 Tbsp Oil
- ✓ 1 Prize Pepper
- ✓ 1 Prize Salt

For the Sauce
- ✓ 50 g Butter
- ✓ 50 g Flour
- ✓ 0.5 Milk
- ✓ 0.5 Soup
- ✓ 1 Msp Nutmeg
- ✓ 1 Prize Pepper
- ✓ 1 Prize Salt

PREPARATION

1. First, the spinach lasagna with béchamel sauce preheat the oven to 200 degrees top/bottom heat and coat an ovenproof dish with oil. Finely dice the feta.

2. Then peel and finely chop the onions and garlic. Sweat both in a bit of oil in a saucepan. Add the still frozen spinach and thaw. Season with salt, pepper, and nutmeg.

3. For the bechamel sauce, melt the butter in a saucepan, then stir in the flour. Gradually pour in the milk and the soup and stir well so that no lumps form. Season with salt, pepper, and nutmeg and simmer for a few minutes.

4. Now alternately layer the sauce, lasagne sheets, spinach, and feta in the baking dish. Start and finish with sauce. Finally, sprinkle the cheese over the lasagne and bake in the oven for 35 minutes.

VEGETARIAN DINNER RECIPES

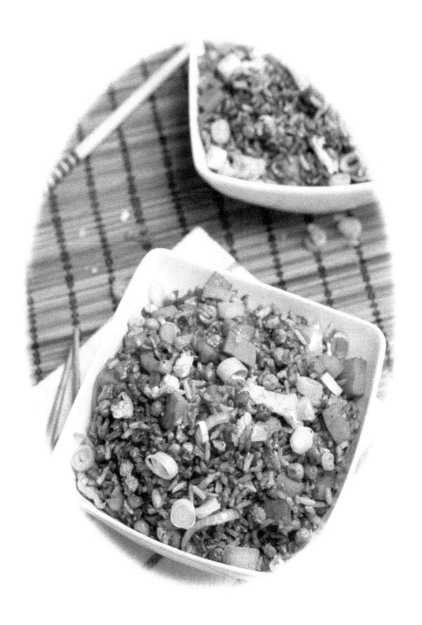

SPAGHETTI WITH MUSHROOM CREAM SAUCE

Servings:4

INGREDIENTS

- ✓ 400 g Mushrooms
- ✓ 2 Tbsp Olive oil
- ✓ 1 Federation Parsley
- ✓ 1 Prize Pepper
- ✓ 270 ml Cream
- ✓ 1 Prize Salt
- ✓ 450 g Spaghetti
- ✓ 1 Pc Oion

PREPARATION

1. The spaghetti is cooked al dente in a large saucepan with boiling salted water for about 8-10 minutes.

2. Meanwhile, rinse off the fresh parsley, shake it dry and chop it finely. Then peel and finely chop the onion. Clean, prepare and slice the fresh mushrooms.

3. Now sauté the onion cubes in a frying pan with a bit of oil for about 5 minutes before stirring in the mushrooms

and frying them for about 3-4 minutes. Deglaze with the white wine and simmer gently over low heat until the mushrooms are soft.

4. Then stir in the cream and season well with salt and pepper.

5. Then pour off the cooked spaghetti, drain well and stir into the sauce. Sprinkle the spaghetti on the mushroom cream sauce with the parsley and serve immediately.

SPAGHETTI WITH BROCCOLI AND NUT SAUCE

Servings1

INGREDIENTS

- ✓ 120 ml Bouillon (vegetables)
- ✓ 150 g Broccoli
- ✓ 60 g Ground hazelnuts
- ✓ 1 Prize Nutmeg
- ✓ 1 Tbsp Olive oil
- ✓ 2 Tbsp Parmesan, grated
- ✓ 1 Prize Pepper
- ✓ 80 ml Cream
- ✓ 1 Prize Salt
- ✓ 150 g Spaghetti
- ✓ 1 Pc Onion

PREPARATION

1. The bouillon is boiled according to the instructions on the package. Peel the fresh onion, chop it finely and sauté in a pan with a bit of oil for about 5 minutes. Deglaze with the stock and cream. Stir in the ground hazelnuts, season

well with salt, pepper, and nutmeg, and slowly reduce to two-thirds.

2. In the meantime, the spaghetti is cooked firm to the bite for about 10 minutes. Wash and prepare the fresh broccoli and cut the florets. Add to the boiling spaghetti in the last 3 minutes or so of the cooking time. Then pour both off and drain well.

3. Put the spaghetti and broccoli in a bowl, mix thoroughly with the sauce and sprinkle with the parmesan. Serve hot immediately.

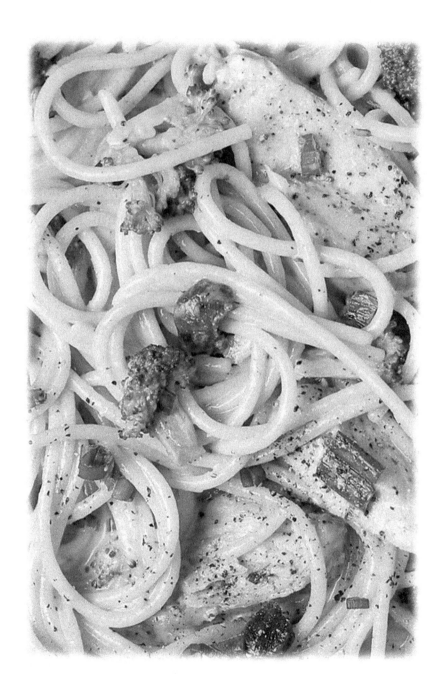

SPAGHETTI WITH A BASIL-LEMON SAUCE

Servings4

INGREDIENTS

- ✓ 3 Tbsp Basil
- ✓ 5 Tbsp Capers
- ✓ 4 Pc Garlic cloves
- ✓ 100 ml Olive oil
- ✓ 1 Prize Pepper
- ✓ 220 ml Cream
- ✓ 1 Prize Salt
- ✓ 450 g Spaghetti
- ✓ 1 Pc Lemon

PREPARATION

1. The spaghetti is cooked al dente in boiling salted water.
2. Meanwhile, peel and finely chop the garlic cloves. Wash the lemon, dry it and grate the peel finely. Then cut in half and squeeze out the juice.
3. The capers are fried in a pan with a bit of oil for about 3 minutes. Then take it out and let it drain on a paper

towel. Sauté the garlic in the pan for about 5 minutes. Add the cream, 1 teaspoon lemon zest, and 1 tablespoon lemon juice, and let it simmer for about 5 minutes. Season well with salt and pepper.

4. Wash the basil leaves, shake dry and finely chop. Drain the spaghetti, mix thoroughly with the sauce, sprinkle with the basil and capers, and arrange plates.

SPAGHETTI WITH AVOCADO AND TOMATO SAUCE

Servings2

INGREDIENTS

- ✓ 1 Pc Avocado
- ✓ 1 Prize Cayenne pepper
- ✓ 1 Pc Clove of garlic
- ✓ 1 Federation Parsley
- ✓ 70 ml Cream
- ✓ 1 Prize Salt
- ✓ 270 g Spaghetti
- ✓ 1 Pc Tomato
- ✓ 2 Tbsp Lemon juice

PREPARATION

1. The spaghetti is cooked al dente in boiling salted water.
2. Meanwhile, cut the fresh avocado in half, remove the stone and spoon out the pulp. Mash it in a bowl with a fork and drizzle with the lemon juice. Wash and chop the firm tomatoes. Peel the garlic and chop it into fine

slithers. Rinse the fresh parsley, shake it dry and chop it just as finely.

3. Heat the avocado mousse with the tomato pieces, parsley, garlic, and cream in a saucepan, but do not bring to the boil. Season well with salt and cayenne pepper.

4. Drain and drain the cooked spaghetti. Mix with the sauce in a saucepan and serve hot immediately.

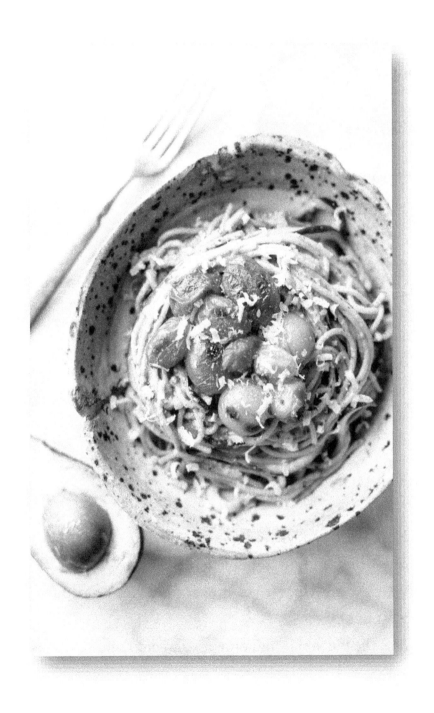

CELERY SALAD WITH ORANGE

Servings4

INGREDIENTS

- ✓ 5 Schb Pineapple
- ✓ 7 Tbsp Vinegar
- ✓ 2 Pc Oranges
- ✓ 350 g Celery bulb
- ✓ 250 ml Water

Dressing
- ✓ 3 Tbsp Mayonnaise
- ✓ 1 Prize Salt and pepper
- ✓ 5 Tbsp Lemon juice

PREPARATION

1. Mix vinegar and saltwater and bring to a boil. Peel the celery bulb and cut it into fine sticks.
2. Pour the hot vinegar water over it and let it steep for a few minutes.
3. Peel the pineapple and oranges and cut them into small pieces.

4. For the dressing, mix the mayonnaise with lemon juice, salt, and pepper.

5. Mix all ingredients and pour the dressing over them.

CELERY CREAM SOUP

Servings4

INGREDIENTS

- ✓ 950 ml Bouillon (vegetables)
- ✓ 1 Tbsp Butter
- ✓ 1 Pc Clove of garlic
- ✓ 1 Prize Nutmeg
- ✓ 1 Tbsp Oil
- ✓ 120 ml Cream
- ✓ 1 Pc Red onion
- ✓ 1 Prize Salt
- ✓ 550 g Celery bulb
- ✓ 120 ml White wine

PREPARATION

1. The bouillon is boiled according to the instructions on the package. Peel and finely chop the red onion and clove of garlic.

2. Peel and dice the fresh celery bulb. Then sauté the prepared ingredients in a saucepan with a bit of oil for about 5 minutes.

3. Deglaze with the bouillon and white wine, cover the pot and simmer gently for about 20 minutes.

4. Then stir in the cream, remove the pan from the stove and puree the soup with the hand blender. If desired, the soup can be strained through a sieve. Season with fleur de sel and nutmeg. The delicious soup is ready.

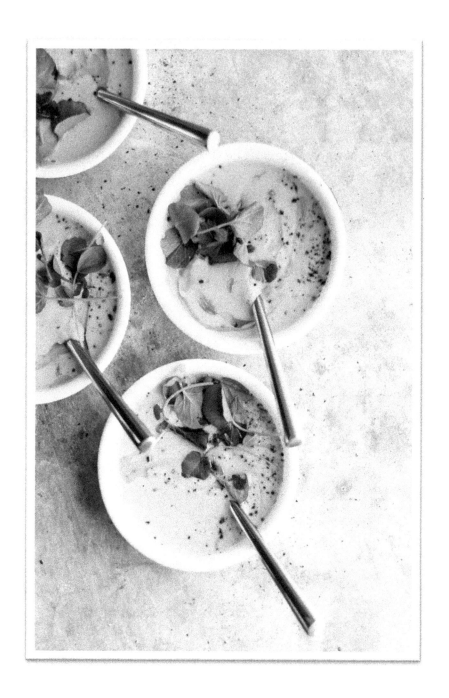

BLACK SALSIFY SOUP

Servings4

INGREDIENTS

- ✓ 750 ml Bouillon (vegetables)
- ✓ 2 Tbsp Butter
- ✓ 1 Pc Potato
- ✓ 230 ml Milk
- ✓ 1 Prize Nutmeg
- ✓ 1 Prize Pepper
- ✓ 150 ml Cream
- ✓ 1 Pc Red Onion
- ✓ 1 Prize Salt
- ✓ 550 g Salsify
- ✓ 1 Between Thyme
- ✓ 1 Pc Vanilla pod
- ✓ 1 Pc Lemon

PREPARATION

1. Black salsify soup the bouillon is boiled according to the instructions on the package. Peel and wash the fresh salsify and cut into bite-sized pieces. Put these in a bowl and drizzle with the lemon juice. Peel and dice the firm potato. Peel and finely chop the red onion.

2. Sauté the onions in a saucepan with a bit of oil for about 5 minutes. Deglaze with the stock and milk. Drain the salsify and add to the pot with the potatoes. Let the whole thing simmer gently. Rinse the thyme sprig and shake dry. Cut the vanilla pod lengthways and scrape out the pulp with the tip of a knife in one go. Mix the vanilla pulp with the pod and thyme into the soup. Season the soup with salt and pepper and simmer for about 25 minutes over medium heat.

3. Then stir in the cream and bring to a boil. Remove the vanilla pod and the sprig of thyme. Remove the pot from the stove and puree it with the soup using a hand blender. Season well with lemon juice and nutmeg. Arrange immediately in soup bowls and serve hot.

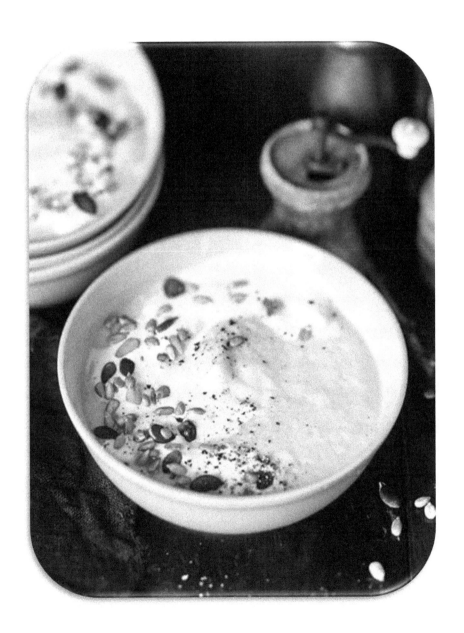

CHIVES - OMELETTE

Servings2

INGREDIENTS

- ✓ 2 Pc Eggs
- ✓ 65 g Flour
- ✓ 100 ml Milk
- ✓ 100 ml Mineral water
- ✓ 1 Shot Oil or butter for the pan
- ✓ 1 Tl Peterli
- ✓ 1 Prize Pepper
- ✓ 1 Prize Salt
- ✓ 0.5 Federation Chives

PREPARATION

1. First, this simple omelet mixes the milk with the mineral water in a bowl, sift in the flour, and stir everything well.
2. Then add the eggs and stir (the order is essential for the consistency of the dough).
3. Wash the herbs (parsley and chives), shake dry, and chop finely. Season the dough with pepper, salt, and spices.

4. Heat some oil or butter in a large pan, pour in half of the batter, and fry the chives omelet until golden brown over medium heat.

5. Pour the remaining batter into the pan, bake the second omelet until golden brown and serve immediately!

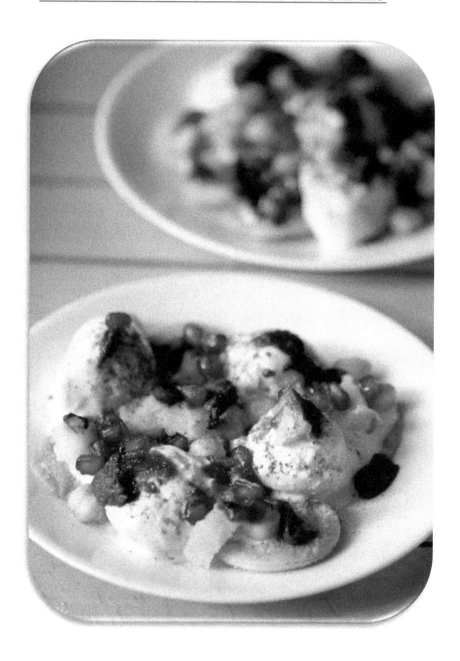

BROCCOLI VEGETABLES

Servings:2

INGREDIENTS

- ✓ 2 Tbsp Butter
- ✓ 2 Pc Garlic cloves
- ✓ 600 g Broccoli
- ✓ 60 g Flaked almonds
- ✓ 70 g Parmesan (grated)
- ✓ 1 Prize Pepper
- ✓ 1 Prize Salt

PREPARATION

1. Briefly toast the almond in a pan without fat.
2. Wash the broccoli, cut into florets, and blanch for a few minutes in a saucepan with salted water.
3. Peel the garlic cloves, cut into slices and sauté with the broccoli in butter. Season with salt and pepper and cook covered for 5 minutes.
4. Sprinkle with the almonds and parmesan and serve immediately.

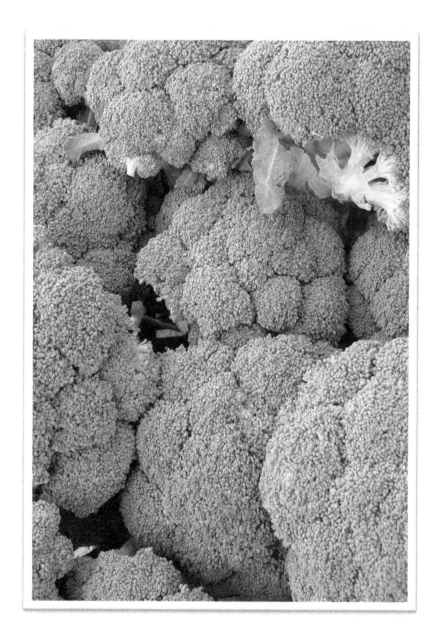

SWEET POTATOES ON THE GRILL

Servings:4

INGREDIENTS

- ✓ 4 Pc Sweet potatoes
- ✓ 1 shot Olive oil
- ✓ 4 Pc Garlic cloves
- ✓ 1 Federation Rosemary
- ✓ 1 Prize Pepper
- ✓ 1 Prize Salt

PREPARATION

1. First, clean and wash the sweet potatoes well and then cut them into small pieces.
2. Prepare 4 sheets of aluminum foil and spread the sweet potatoes on top. Then drizzle with olive oil and season with salt and pepper. Put a peeled clove of garlic and a sprig of rosemary in each packet.
3. Wrap everything up and place it on the grill for about 45 minutes.

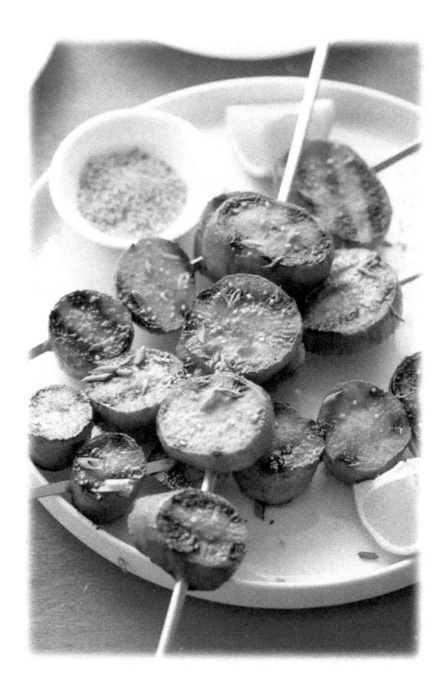

OVEN VEGETABLES ON THE TRAY

Servings:4

INGREDIENTS

- ✓ 1 kg Potatoes
- ✓ 5 Tbsp Olive oil
- ✓ 1 Prize Salt
- ✓ 1 Prize Pepper from the grinder)
- ✓ 2 Pc Red peppers
- ✓ 1 Pc Zucchini
- ✓ 1 Pc Eggplant
- ✓ 6 Pc Rosemary sprigs

PREPARATION

1. The oven vegetables on the baking sheet, first preheat the oven to 200 degrees top/bottom heat and coat a baking sheet with a bit of oil. Peel and quarter the potatoes. Now distribute this on the baking sheet and put it in the oven for half an hour.

2. In the meantime, wash and clean the zucchini, bell pepper, and aubergine and cut them into bite-sized pieces.

3. After half an hour, add the vegetables to the potatoes. Season with salt and pepper and drizzle with oil. Spread the rosemary sprigs on top.

4. Now put the vegetables back in the oven and cook for another 30 minutes.

PASTA WITH GORGONZOLA SAUCE

Servings:2

INGREDIENTS

- ✓ 250 g Pasta
- ✓ 1 Pc Onion
- ✓ 1 Tbsp Oil
- ✓ 0.125 l Soup
- ✓ 150 g Gorgonzola
- ✓ 0.5 Cups Whipped cream
- ✓ 1 Prize Pepper
- ✓ 1 Prize Salt

PREPARATION

1. For the pasta with Gorgonzola sauce, first, peel and finely chop the onion. Sauté in a saucepan with a bit of oil. Cut the cheese into small pieces.
2. In the meantime, cook the noodles in a pan with salted water until they are firm to the bite, strain, and keep warm.
3. Pour on the onion pieces with some soup and add the cheese. Let everything simmer gently until the cheese

has melted. Now pour in the cream and bring to the boil again briefly.

4. Season the sauce with salt and pepper and pour over the pasta.

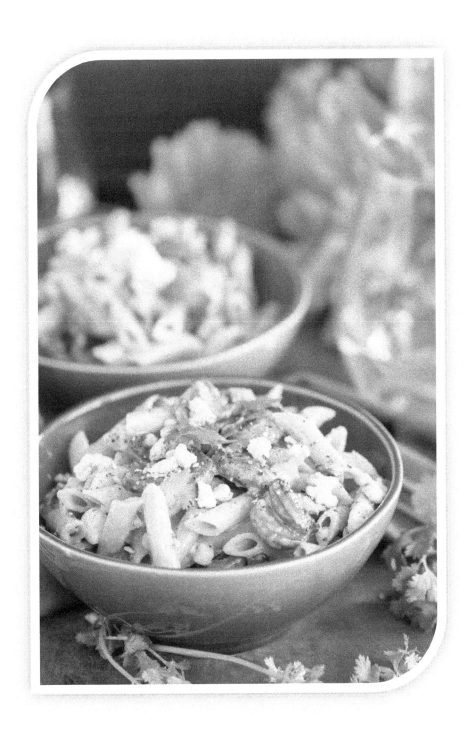

ORIENTAL LENTIL SOUP

Servings:4

INGREDIENTS

- ✓ 1 Prize Salt
- ✓ 1 Pc Onion
- ✓ 3 Pc Carrots
- ✓ 1 PcChilli pepper (red)
- ✓ 200 g Lentils (red)
- ✓ 1 Tbsp Butter
- ✓ 1 Tbsp Turmeric
- ✓ 1 Tl Curry
- ✓ Vegetable Soup
- ✓ 1 Federation Corinander
- ✓ 2 Tbsp Lime juice
- ✓ 1 Cups Yogurt

PREPARATION

1. For the oriental lentil soup, first, peel the onion and carrots and grate them finely. Halve the chili lengthways, core, and finely chop. Put the lentils in a colander and rinse briefly under cold water.

2. Heat the butter in a pan. Sauté the onion, carrots, and chili pepper in it. Then add the turmeric, curry powder, soup, and lentils. Cover and cook the soup for about 15 minutes until the lentils are soft.

3. In the meantime, wash and finely chop the coriander. Season the soup with salt and a little lime juice.

4. Stir the yogurt in a bowl until smooth and lightly season with salt. To serve, bring the soup to the boil again and stir in the coriander. Arrange in preheated plates and add 1 tablespoon of yogurt to the soup.

SPICY EGG SPREAD

Servings:6

INGREDIENTS

- ✓ 6 Pc Hard-boiled eggs
- ✓ 100 ml Mayonnaise
- ✓ 1 Prize Salt
- ✓ 1 Prize Pepper
- ✓ 1 Prize Curry powder

PREPARATION

1. The shells are removed from the hard-boiled eggs. Then they are roughly chopped and mixed well with mayonnaise.
2. The spread is seasoned to taste with salt, pepper, and curry powder. Decorate with roughly chopped chives.

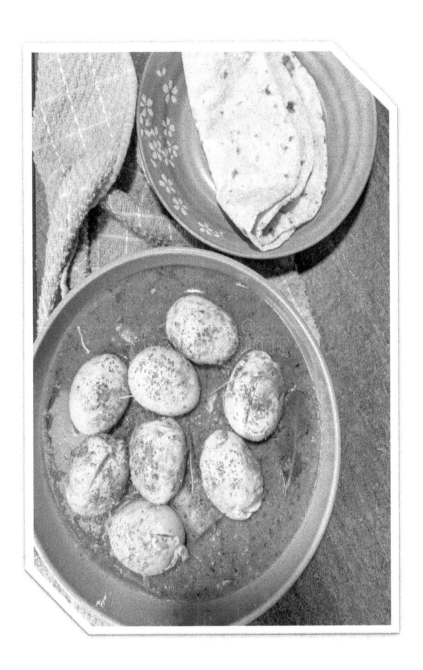

FALAFEL WITH CHICKPEA FLOUR

Servings:4

INGREDIENTS

- ✓ 120 g Chickpea flour
- ✓ 1 Msp Cumin
- ✓ 2 Tbsp Parsley (frozen)
- ✓ 1 Pc Onion
- ✓ 3 Pc Garlic cloves
- ✓ 0.5 Tl baking powder
- ✓ 1 Tl Salt
- ✓ 150 ml Water
- ✓ 1 Tbsp Olive oil

PREPARATION

1. For falafel with chickpea flour, first, peel and finely chop the onion and garlic. Then mix with the flour, baking powder, parsley, cumin, and salt in a bowl.

2. Bring the water to a boil in a saucepan and slowly stir into the flour mixture. Finally, mix in the oil and lemon juice and let the mixture steep for 15 minutes.

3. Then shape small patties with wet hands. Heat the oil in a deep pan and bake the cakes until golden on both sides.

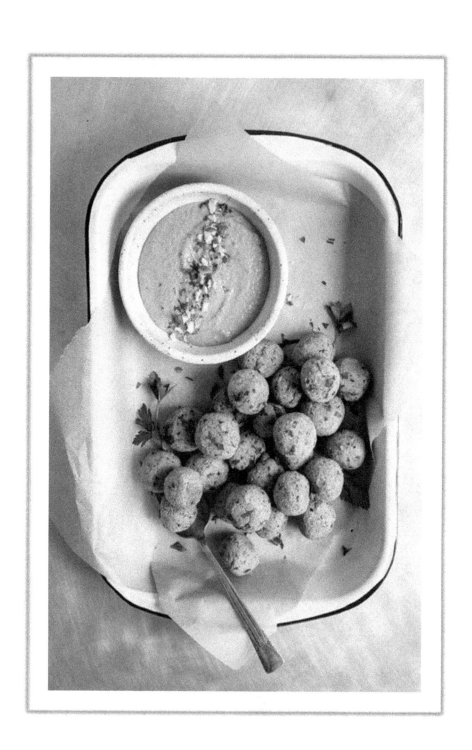

FIRE PATCH

Servings:4

INGREDIENTS

- ✓ 500 g Rye flour
- ✓ 500 g Wheat flour
- ✓ 250 ml Warm water
- ✓ 8 Tbsp Oil
- ✓ 1 Tl Salt
- ✓ 1 TL Sugar
- ✓ 1 Pk Germ

PREPARATION

1. For the fire stains, mix yeast with sugar, add flour, water, milk, oil, and salt. Knead into a dough with the mixer, let the dough rise in a warm place for 30 minutes.
2. Then roll out thin flatbreads and bake them in a hot, coated pan without fat. The flatbread must form bubbles.

STRUDEL WITH VEGETABLES

Servings:4

INGREDIENTS

- ✓ 1 Pk Strudel dough (according to the basic recipe or ready)
- ✓ 700 g Vegetables - frozen
- ✓ 1 Cups Creme fraiche with herbs
- ✓ 2 Pc Garlic cloves
- ✓ 50 g Cheese (grated)
- ✓ 1 Prize Pepper
- ✓ 1 Prize Salt

PREPARATION

1. For the strudel dough with vegetables, first, let the vegetables thaw a little. Preheat the oven to 200 degrees hot air and line a baking sheet with parchment paper. Roll out the dough on the baking sheet.
2. Peel the garlic and squeeze it into a bowl. Mix with the vegetables and creme fraiche and season with salt and pepper.

3. Spread the vegetable mixture on the dough and roll-up. Press the ends firmly and brush the strudel with water.
4. Then sprinkle with cheese and bake in the oven for about 30 minutes until golden brown.

VEGETARIAN DESSERT RECIPES

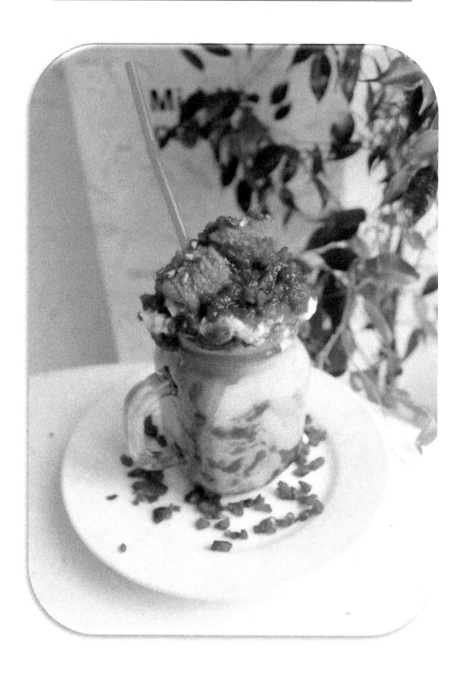

REFRESHING CUPCAKES WITH A STRAWBERRY CREAM TOPPING

Servings:12

INGREDIENTS

- ✓ 2 Pc Eggs
- ✓ 100 g Sugar
- ✓ 100 ml Oil
- ✓ 100 ml Orange juice
- ✓ 0.5 Pc Lemon, squeezed
- ✓ 150 g Flour
- ✓ 1 TL Baking powder
- ✓ 50 g Almonds, chopped

for the topping
- ✓ 250 g Strawberries
- ✓ 200 ml Whipped cream
- ✓ 1 Pk Cream stiffener
- ✓ 1 Pk Vanilla sugar
- ✓ 125 g Quark (lean

PREPARATION

1. Preheat the oven to 175 ° C and line the muffin tin with paper liners.
2. Beat eggs and sugar until creamy, then add oil, orange, and lemon juice.
3. Now stir in the baking powder and flour quickly into the butter mixture and then lift the almonds into the dough.
4. Distribute the batter evenly in the molds and bake the cakes on the middle rack for about 25 minutes.
5. Put one strawberry aside for each cupcake and puree the rest. Then add the curd cheese and stir everything into a smooth mass.
6. Beat the whipped cream with the cream stiffener and vanilla sugar until stiff and fold it into the strawberry curd mixture.
7. Put the finished cream in a piping bag and garnish the cooled cupcakes with it. Finally, put the strawberries on the cream.

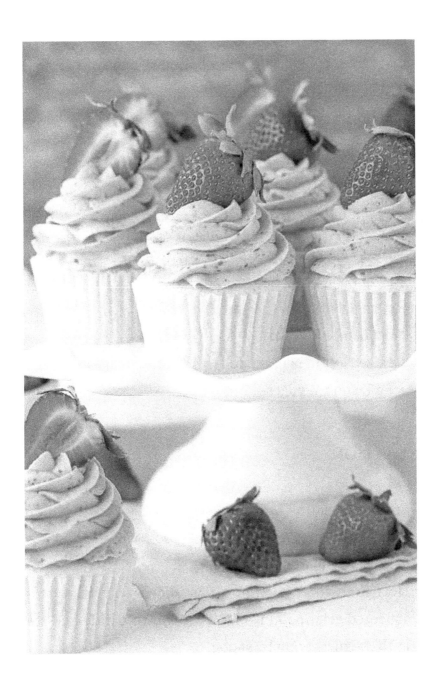

YOGURT LEMON CREAM

Servings:

INGREDIENTS

- ✓ 4 Bl Gelatin (white)
- ✓ 150 g Greek plain yogurt
- ✓ 1 Tl Lemon peel (finely grated)
- ✓ 2 Tbsp Fine granulated sugar
- ✓ 3 Tbsp Lemon juice
- ✓ 225 ml Obers
- ✓ 4 Pc Lemon wedges
- ✓ 4 Prize Lemon peel (grated)
- ✓ 4 Pc Lemon Wedges

PREPARATION

1. Soak the gelatine in cold water. Mix the Greek natural yogurt with the sugar and the teaspoon of lemon zest and let it steep for 10 minutes.

2. Heat the lemon juice in a pan and dissolve the well-squeezed gelatine in it - let it cool down a little and stir in the yogurt spoon by spoon.

3. Beat the cream until stiff and fold it carefully into the yogurt mixture.
4. Fill the lemon cream into glasses or lemon halves and refrigerate for at least 2 hours.
5. Decorate the lemon cream with lemon wedges and grated lemon zest and serve.

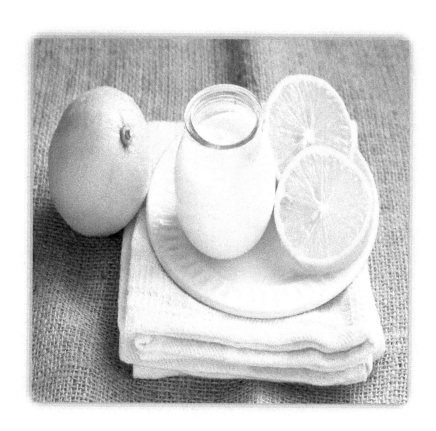

RODON CAKE

Servings:12

INGREDIENTS

- ✓ 1 Pk Baking powder
- ✓ 230 g Butter
- ✓ 1 Tbsp Butter, for greasing
- ✓ 3 Pc Eggs
- ✓ 3 Tbsp Cocoa powder
- ✓ 450 g Flour
- ✓ 2 Tbsp Flour, for sprinkling
- ✓ 7 Tbsp Milk
- ✓ 220 g Sugar

PREPARATION

1. Beat the butter and sugar until foamy and slowly stir in the eggs.
2. Mix the flour with the baking powder and stir into the butter, egg mixture. Let the milk flow in slowly.
3. Grease the loaf pan and dust with flour. First, fill in half of the dough, then mix the other half of the dough with cocoa powder and finish filling the loaf pan.

4. To create a lovely pattern, pull through the dough with a fork.

5. Preheat the oven, bake the cake at 180 degrees for 60 minutes, then the cake has to cool down.

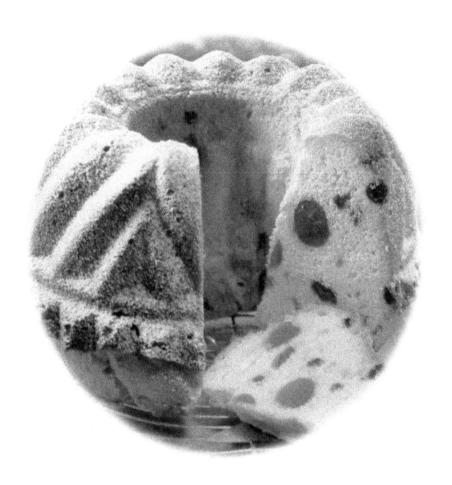

CHESTNUT TERRINE

Servings:10

INGREDIENTS

- ✓ 1 Pk Lady fingers (ladyfingers)
- ✓ 1 Bl Gelatin
- ✓ 0.25 l Coffee (black, sugared)
- ✓ 500 g Chestnut puree
- ✓ 1 cl Rum or orange liqueur
- ✓ 0.125 l Whipped cream (whipped)
- ✓ 1 Pk Vanilla sugar
- ✓ 50 g Icing sugar

PREPARATION

1. Mix the chestnut mixture with icing sugar and rum and stir until smooth.
2. Fold in the whipped cream and mix in the soaked - warmed gelatine.
3. Line a mold with cling film, spread a thin layer of white cream, and line the biscuits dipped in coffee with it.
4. Then fill the tub in layers alternately with chestnut paste and ladyfingers.

5. Finally, smooth it out with white cream and refrigerate, preferably overnight.

FRUCHTIKUS SLICES

Servings:12

INGREDIENTS

- ✓ 5 Pc Egg yolk
- ✓ 5 Pc Egg white
- ✓ 250 g Sugar
- ✓ 125 ml Oil
- ✓ 125 ml Water
- ✓ 200 g Flour
- ✓ 40 g Cocoa powder
- ✓ 1 Pk Baking powder

for the cream

- ✓ 3 Pk Creme fraiche Cheese
- ✓ 500 ml Whipped cream
- ✓ 7 Tbsp Sugar
- ✓ 8 Bl Gelatin
- ✓ 500 g Peaches (pureed, can, or fresh)

PREPARATION

1. In a bowl, beat the yolks, sugar, oil, and water until frothy. Mix the flour with the baking powder and fold into the yolk mass.

2. Beat the egg whites very stiffly and then fold them into the yolk mass with the cocoa. Spread on a baking sheet lined with baking paper and bake in the preheated oven at 180 ° C for approx. 25-30 minutes with top and bottom heat. Then let the cake cool down.

3. For the cream: Mix the creme fraiche with the sugar. Then fold in the whipped cream.

4. For the glaze: puree the peaches and add the melted gelatine.

5. Now the cream is applied to the cooled cake. Then the peach glaze comes over the cream. Put everything in a cool place for approx. 2 hours, then cut into the desired pieces.

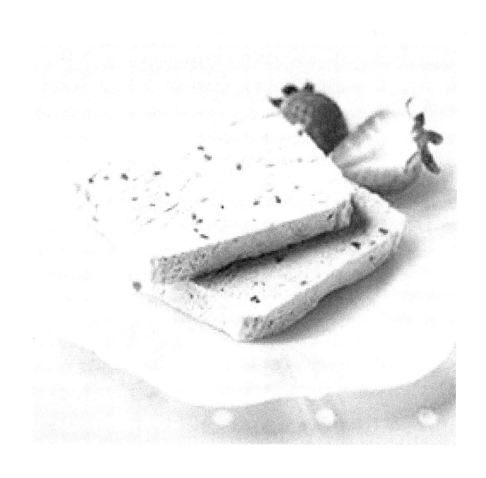

COCONUT BISCUIT (PALEO)

Servings:1

INGREDIENTS

- ✓ 1 Pk Baking powder
- ✓ 3 Pc Yolk
- ✓ 3 Pc Egg white
- ✓ 100 g Honey
- ✓ 50 g Coconut flakes
- ✓ 3 Tbsp Coconut flour
- ✓ 100 ml Coconut milk
- ✓ 4 Tbsp Water

PREPARATION

1. Stir/mix yolks, honey, and water until foamy. Add coconut flour, baking powder, coconut flakes, and coconut milk.
2. Beat egg whites until stiff. Fold the egg whites into the rest of the mixture. Preheat the oven to 180 degrees bake until golden for 20 minutes.

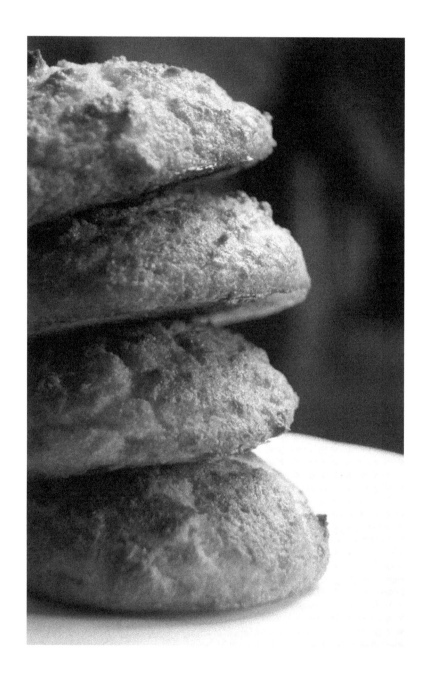

BEETROOT - CHOCOLATE BROWNIES (PALEO)

Servings:20

INGREDIENTS

- ✓ 3 Pc Eggs
- ✓ 300 g Beetroot
- ✓ 5 Tbsp Honey
- ✓ 3 Tbsp Coconut flour
- ✓ 250 g Dark chocolate (85%)
- ✓ 2 Tbsp Cocoa powder
- ✓ 100 g Coconut oil
- ✓ 100 g Grated hazelnuts
- ✓ 2 Tbsp Coarsely chopped hazelnuts
- ✓ 1 Prize Pepper
- ✓ 1 Tl Baking powder

PREPARATION

1. Peel and cook beets until cooked through. Then puree with the hand blender or the food processor.
2. Add eggs, honey, cocoa powder, and pepper to the beetroot.

3. Heat 150 grams of the chocolate with coconut oil and let it melt. Roughly chop 100 grams of the chocolate.

4. Add liquid chocolate to the beet paste. Stir in baking powder, nuts, and coconut flour.

5. Finally, stir the chocolate pieces into the mass. Mass at 180 degrees for 40 minutes in the preheated oven.

6. ATTENTION: Take out of the oven after 40 minutes and let cool in the mold. Only then lift it out of the mold together with the baking paper and cut. (Even if the curiosity is great, really wait until it has completely cooled down!).

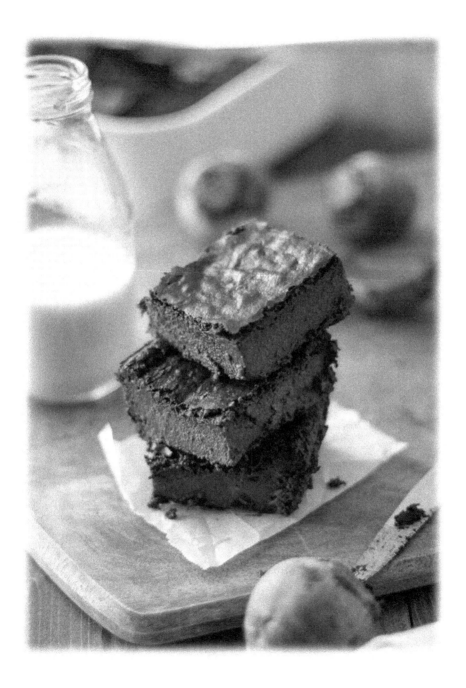

PANNA COTTA WITH RASPBERRIES

Servings:4

INGREDIENTS

- ✓ 0.06 l Milk
- ✓ 40 g Sugar
- ✓ 0.5 Tbsp Vanilla sugar
- ✓ 0.25 l Whipped cream
- ✓ 8 Bl Gelatin
- ✓ 120 g Raspberries
- ✓ 5 g Sugar
- ✓ 4 Bl Mint

PREPARATION

1. Bring the milk, sugar, and vanilla sugar to the boil in a saucepan, then add the whipped cream and bring to the boil again.
2. Soak 4 sheets of gelatine in water, squeeze out and dissolve in 2 tablespoons of water. Add gelatin to the cooked mass and pour into suitable glasses that have been rinsed once.

3. Strain the raspberries, then bring to the boil with sugar and add the dissolved gelatin. Then pour the raspberry sauce onto the panna cotta and place in the fridge for about 1.5 hours.

4. Refine with fresh whole raspberry pieces and mint leaves before serving.

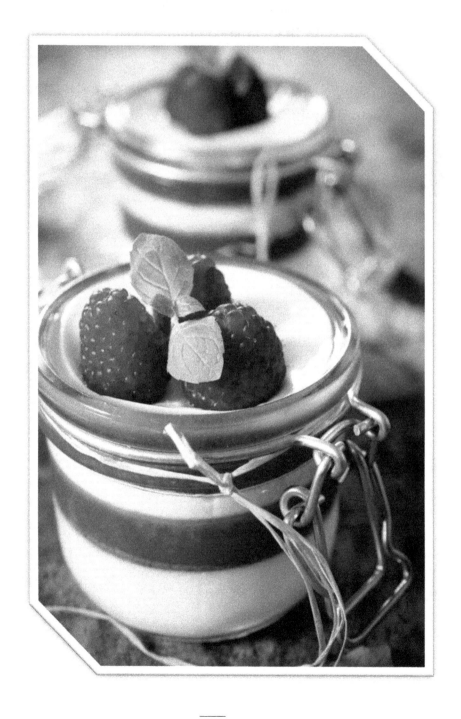

CONCLUSION

The consumption of meat has a significant impact on the environment and thus also on climate change. Because more than 14% of all greenhouse gas emissions are due to meat production - and the associated animal husbandry. This is one of the advantages of a vegetarian diet, but it also has disadvantages.

BENEFITS OF A VEGETARIAN DIET
Those who follow a vegetarian diet are also committed to the environment.

INCREASED WELL-BEING:
In addition to the benefits for the environment and animals, a well-planned vegetarian diet also positively influences physical and mental well-being.

A VEGETARIAN DIET IS HEALTHY:

According to studies, vegetarians have above-average health. Of course, the prerequisite for this is that you have a varied and balanced vegetarian diet despite not eating meat and fish.

HEALTH BENEFITS:

With a balanced diet, vegetarians usually have
Better blood pressure readings
A healthier body weight
Are less likely to develop diabetes
Risk factors from processed and red meat are eliminated. These can promote the development of cancer or cardiovascular diseases.
Vegetarian diet - the disadvantages
At the same time, however, a meat- and fish-free diet also harbors risks.
Undersupply: Due to the lack of supply,
there may be an undersupply of some essential nutrients, vitamins and trace elements.

DEFICIENCY:

There is a deficiency in vegetarians Vitamin B12, iron, iodine, calcium, or zinc are not uncommon.

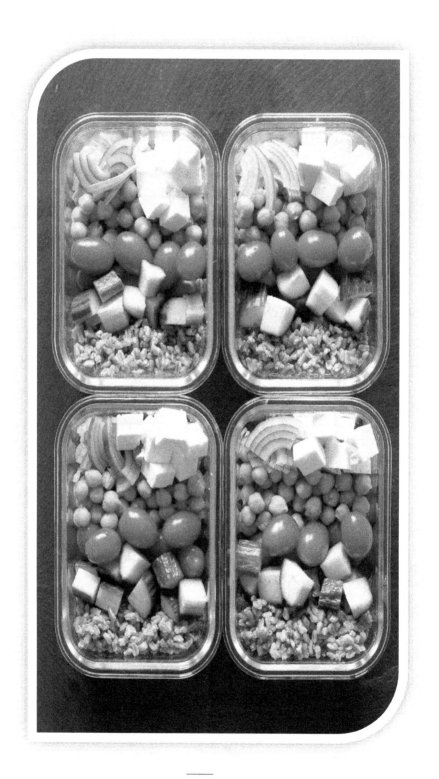

CPSIA information can be obtained
at www.ICGtesting.com
Printed in the USA
LVHW081815010621
689062LV00015B/1790

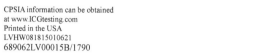

9 781914 121760